SIMPLE FITNESS
A NO NONSENSE APPROACH

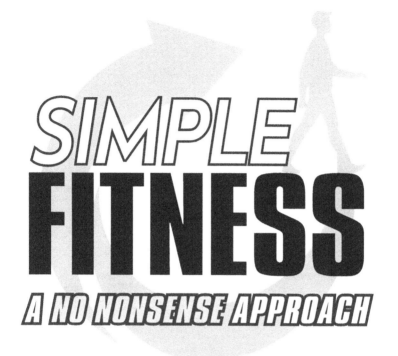

SIMPLE FITNESS
A NO NONSENSE APPROACH

ROBERT MACDOUGALL
AKA "COACH MAC"

Copyright © 2023 Robert MacDougall.

All rights reserved. No part of this book may be used or reproduced in any manner whatsoever without written permission of the author. Published 2023.

Printed in the United States of America.

ISBN: 978-1-63385-506-9
Library of Congress Control Number: 2023920805

Published by
Word Association Publishers
205 Fifth Avenue
Tarentum, Pennsylvania 15084

www.wordassociation.com
1.800.827.7903

PREFACE

When Gutzon Borglum set out to create Mount Rushmore National Monument, his task was simple: Cut away everything from the mountain face that didn't look like a president. In practice, of course, jackhammering and blasting rocks out of the cliff to create those faces was a monumentally difficult project that took decades. Clearly "easy" is not a synonym for "simple."

Take, for example, getting or remaining physically fit. It is indisputable that a person who eats moderate amounts of food and exercises regularly will maintain a pretty good level of fitness. It is also axiomatic that a person who wants to lose weight and have a better level of fitness would be able to achieve his/her goals if he/she ate less and exercised more. It is all very simple. Yet, for many people, actually doing those two things is decidedly difficult. So, what I will try to do is describe some of the most effective ways I have found to "eat less and exercise more" and assure you that you don't have to turn your life inside out to make great progress and be more fit and probably happier than you have been in quite a while.

Unlike any other book I have written, this one can be devoured in thirty minutes. Why not give it a go and take at least some of the advice it offers, make the simple adjustments in your life that it prescribes, and then go your merry way?

CONTENTS

INTRODUCTION: WHY FITNESS?....................1
CHAPTER I: EAT LESS 5
CHAPTER II: WALK MORE 19
CONCLUSION: IS THAT IT? 29
APPENDIX A 35
APPENDIX B 37

INTRODUCTION

THE PHYSICAL FITNESS CONUNDRUM

Every day I interact with or observe many people who are not happy with their health or physical appearance. They must take statin drugs to deal with high cholesterol; they are on one of several blood pressure medications; they have a stomach that looks like they just swallowed a bowling ball or they have a roll of fat that hangs over their belt. Even worse, they are constantly thinking negative thoughts such as: "Do I look fat?" or "Why am I so tired all the time?" Many people have tried programs that promise to make them feel better and see themselves more positively, and sometimes the promise is fulfilled . . . briefly. Then, the backsliding begins and they are right back where they started. The problems with the programs they have followed is usually that they are too complicated and/or require too much of a change in the lifestyle they would normally choose to lead.

If any of the above descriptions applies to you, or if you are concerned that some of them soon will, then you might want to consider some of the health concepts that I am about to recommend. As you will see, my plan is very simple . . . not necessarily easy, at least at first, but simple. Once you adjust to the concepts and the rhythms of it, you will see that it is the kind of lifestyle you can maintain until you pass into eternity and become liberated from all bodily concerns. If you follow my advice, even partially, you will not have to buy anything or do any weird things.

Now, I will tell you a few basic facts about me that might help you give a little more credence to what I say in these pages. When I graduated from high school in 1962, I was 5'10" tall and weighed 155 pounds; my pants were 32" waist. Today I am 5'8" tall and weigh 155 pounds; my pants are 32" waist. Gravity has taken a toll on me, but I have never gained an ounce of weight or an inch of belly fat. I tell you these numbers just to convince you that I know what I am talking about. To achieve these numbers (while rarely looking at a scale), I have "walked the walk" so to speak and, I hasten to add, I have thoroughly enjoyed life the entire time. The only times I have been a bit unhappy (excluding, of course, times of deaths and illnesses) are those times when I have eaten too much and felt sluggishly stuffed, and those times when I have been laid up and unable to go for a bracing run or walk.

I tell you these things at the risk of being thought a braggard. I am far from prideful about my health and weight. I know very well that it is only through God's grace that I have been healthy enough, lucky enough, and free enough, to eat and exercise as I wish. I have often thought of the friends I have had who were stuck in wheelchairs or otherwise restricted and would have given every penny they owned just to be able to do what I was doing for one day.

I am very aware that there is nothing new in what I am about to tell you. It has always been a cause of great mirth to me – and sometimes annoyed anger – when I read or hear on the news that "recent studies" have shown that the key to weight control and good health is diet and exercise. NO KIDDING!! How many times does that have to be proved?? So, in the pages that follow, I will be telling you nothing new or astounding. All I hope to do is give you, in unvarnished terms, my prescription for how to achieve optimal results from your diet and your exercise routines. The theme will be: Keep it simple! Do not overcomplicate things with burdensome theories, measurements, time schedules, and anything else that will weigh down your daily life and cause you to give up on the whole fitness thing as an annoyance you can do without.

Finally, I want this book to be a frontal assault on the way we think about wellness and healthcare these days. The current mindset seems to be that scientists study the various diseases and maladies and try to develop medications to deal with them. They are even starting to prescribe medications to control childhood obesity! I believe this is a misguided approach! We should spend much more of our efforts on keeping people from getting ill in the first place and helping them stay fit enough to fight off the maladies that attack them if they do become ill. A major component of the fight against the Covid virus that was completely ignored was the need to keep everyone in the world as fit as possible. Rather than quarantining all the healthy people, the governments should have been encouraging everyone to get out, exercise and control their weight. Instead, they forced people to stay in their homes . . . and, presumably, get fat and out of shape! I'll never forget the scene of the police officer on a jet ski arresting a lone surfer in California! During the pandemic restrictions, people everywhere got depressed, fatter and much more likely to get severely ill.

I would really like to see the next President of the United States, no matter who it is, strongly advocate a program of physical fitness. The nation is due for such a thing. In 1903 President Theodore Roosevelt advocated "the strenuous life" and urged Americans to go out into the great outdoors and exercise. Sixty years later, in 1963, President Kennedy heartily encouraged fitness and even advocated fifty-mile hikes, something I tried myself that year. (No, I failed!) Now, another sixty years have passed and it's time for another American president to urgently encourage fitness. It's more than just time for it; the country desperately needs it!

With this book I am trying to do my small part to get people to eat less and exercise more. I am not the president and I only have modest credentials to convince people to follow my advice. But I hope you will find my advice logical and doable and that you will be inspired enough to follow it and, even more important, stick with it. This is a plan for the long term.

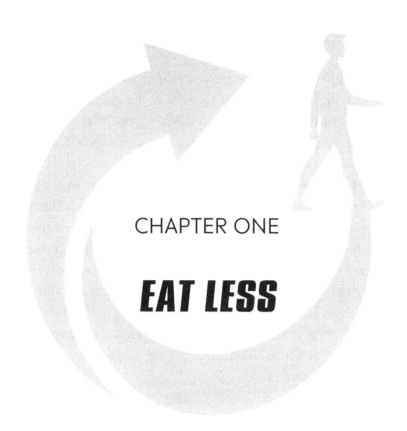

CHAPTER ONE

EAT LESS

This diet plan will begin by saying something that other diet plans will never say:

Diet plans are unwieldy and ultimately useless. I've seen people carefully measure exact amounts of certain foods they are "allowed" to eat under their new "guaranteed to cut inches off your waist" plans and dutifully follow every minute detail, right down to the bedtime snack they are allowed to have. They have almost always achieved limited or no success and then have given up the entire thing as too cumbersome and annoying to continue. Any diet plans that require you to measure everything you put into your mouth, or eat only certain foods (e.g. the grapefruit diet, the "no carb" diet, etc.), or do anything else that deviates almost entirely from your ordinary life, is guaranteed to fail because *you will get sick of it.*

Then there are the weight loss programs that ship you the food all ready to stick into the oven or microwave. Those plans are convenient, but the food they send you is so minimal that you will probably "supplement" it even though you are not supposed to. And then . . . the bills come. Do you really want to send huge quantities of cash to those unknown people you have put in charge of what you eat?

My diet plan is so simple it really cannot be called a plan. It is stated in RULE NUMBER ONE for weight control and good health: EAT LESS!!

That's all there is to it. Eat pretty much what you want, just don't eat so much of it. It *is* important to eat as little sugar and white flour as possible, but beyond that, if you have a weight problem it is almost certainly because you eat too much and/or too often. So, the question arises, "How do I change my lifestyle to stop eating too much?

Any diet plan that requires you to measure everything or eat only certain foods is guaranteed to fail!

The first step is to shake off the idea that you live to eat. If you feel that one of life's greatest pleasures is eating, if you are constantly dreaming about the next delicious thing you are going to put into your mouth, if the very thought of eating certain foods is positively orgasmic, then you need a major thought overhaul. You need to think of food not as an experience, but as *fuel* for your body's engine. Determine which foods work best in your engine and focus on those, not for the taste experience but for the fuel and health benefits they will give you. Think of foods that are clearly *bad* for you – such as sugar – as poison and *eliminate them* from your sight! Long ago I developed a habit of looking at such things as donuts, sodas and candy bars and thinking, "They are laced with rattlesnake venom!" That thought makes it easy for me to turn them down.

The second step is to remind yourself, as often as necessary, that the goal of each meal is to fuel up with food that will give you energy and help you fight off illness. It is NOT to stuff yourself with food that will only make you uncomfortable for hours. Even if you were brought up "old school" and told to eat everything on your plate, shake off that thought and stop eating when you feel full, or know that you have had enough. Remember, it is better that excess food go into the garbage, or better yet, into a container for tomorrow, than onto your waistline.

The third step is to decide exactly which foods you will eat as your regular diet and which you will avoid entirely. Then, stock up on the good stuff and get rid of the bad. Lay in large quantities of vegetables, fruit, oatmeal, lean meat – the things I will discuss a bit later -- and throw out all the bad, gunky stuff and never buy any of it again. It is very important not to have any "bad" food in the house at all. I am as undisciplined as anyone about not being able to resist sugary foods; I would devour an entire sleeve of chocolate chip cookies in one sitting if I couldn't stop myself and, with that particular cookie, I probably *couldn't* stop myself! So, I just don't have them around; I never buy them. *Resist the temptation in the store and you won't have to resist the temptation at home!*

The fourth and final step is to start eating the right foods on a regular schedule and – this is the crucial part – decide that you *love it*! I am a firm believer in the concept that love is a decision; we can *decide* to love something. So, make that decision. I will make it easier for you by asking this question: Don't you *have to* love something that keeps you healthy and makes you look and feel good?

So, let's get down to it. What are the foods that will give you good health and will make you feel good? I'll start each of the meals with what I usually eat for that meal. Now, to make sure we understand each other, I can readily see how you might despise my food choices, and that is fine. One woman told me she can't stand oatmeal; it reminds her of wallpaper paste! It *does,* kind of, and after she said that it took me a few days to get back to eating it again. But, that's not a reason to abandon my program. Go to one of the other choices. I will suggest several for each meal and, for variety, you might want to vary your choices each day rather than do as I do and eat pretty much the same thing at each meal every day. The key concept is: eat pretty much what you like, *just not too much of it!*

BREAKFAST:

My Usual: OATMEAL (a large bowl, a half a cup of oats before cooking). I have devoured a large bowl of oatmeal nearly every morning for the last fifty years. I also have a bowl of blueberries and a banana. There are several other fruits that would be good: strawberries, peaches, raspberries, and I sometimes top the oatmeal with almonds or walnuts. If you absolutely cannot abide oatmeal without a sweetener on top, use honey. It tastes great and provides good nutrition. Do *not c*over your oatmeal with sugar, white or brown, or with maple syrup.

The oatmeal helps lower cholesterol, and the blueberries and bananas are packed with antioxidants which strengthen your immune system. This breakfast is very filling and, if I have a busy schedule ahead, it can keep me going all day – no need to stop for lunch -- the one meal each day that is rather superfluous. More on this later, but as a foreshadow, I think lunch is a good reason to get together with people, but nutritionally it can be a disaster.

I also take a 500 mg zinc tablet at breakfast. Zinc also fortifies your immune system and I have found I have been free of even mild colds for the year I have been taking it. At the risk of getting political I will reiterate what I said in the Introduction: If the various governments (state, federal, other countries) had encouraged people to get out and exercise and to take zinc and eat a healthy diet like the one I am setting forth here, the Covid epidemic might have been less severe. We will never know, but we DO know that locking people down has had so many bad effects – including deaths from things other than Covid – that it seems very likely that an open air, diet and exercise program would have, at the very least, ameliorated the Covid scourge, and maybe we would have emerged from the nightmare with a fitter and more mentally healthy population.

Actually, it's not too late. If everyone followed the recommendations in this book, we would have a good running start toward the way we would handle the next pandemic and people would be healthier and less likely to sicken and die.

Now for those of you who cannot get past the "wallpaper paste" simile, I'll suggest some breakfasts other than oatmeal that would be good for health and weight control.

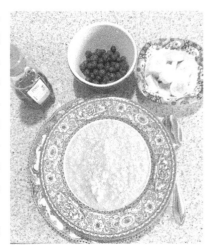

Coach Mac's breakfast of champions: Oatmeal, blueberries and a banana.

BUT FIRST, **A MAJOR WARNING**: Donuts, Croissants, coffee cakes – pretty much everything made with flour and sugar are all poison! THEY ARE LACED WITH RATTLESNAKE VENOM. Do not buy them! Do not eat them . . . in the morning . . . or EVER! They are not part of a decent breakfast, or any other meal.

Also, do not substitute processed cereals for the oatmeal. Other kinds of cooked cereals such as Cream of Wheat or Wheatena are good, but cold cereals such as Corn Flakes, Wheaties, Cheerios, and sixty-five other names, are all loaded with sugar. Avoid them! I hate to admit that as a young boy I sprinkled a spoonful or two of white sugar on my Wheaties every morning. It's a good thing I was a very active child or I would have emerged from childhood a big fat guy.

Finally -- and this I must put in the strongest possible language -- do NOT drink sodas or juices that have sugar in them. These are not laced with rattlesnake venom; they ARE rattlesnake venom. Many studies have proved that the rise in obesity has directly correlated with the rise in the consumption of soft drinks and juices that are loaded with sugar. The "diet" sodas might be a less egregious substitute, but I also try to avoid those because of the questionable sugar substitutes that are in them. The best choice is to simply drink "Adam's Ale," better known as water. If you are slightly masochistic and must have the tingle in your mouth that carbonation offers, try soda water. Really . . . it's not bad just by itself.

Now, I'm not a food Nazi about this -- or any food, really – so, if you absolutely cannot start your day without your bagel and cream cheese or your English muffin topped with butter and jam, then "have at it." In college I had a roommate from New York City who could not start the day without his bagel and lox. But, limit this kind of food -- indeed, limit the *portion* of *any* food -- and at least try to eat the breakfast and other meals that I will recommend.

Other Good Breakfasts: A couple of eggs (any style) and a couple of slices of toast with butter and/or jam is a very good breakfast. I usually don't want to take the time to prepare it when I have to rush out the door to work, but it is perfectly fine nutritionally. A couple of strips of bacon, well cooked and drained, is very tasty and is OK occasionally, but I wouldn't have it every day. By the way, avoid drinking a glass of orange juice each morning. It is loaded with sugar and, if you are concerned about getting enough vitamin C, take a pill along with your Zinc.

Pancakes! One of my favorite foods and I've always enjoyed eating a stack of them with maple syrup and butter dripping down the sides. Having "flapjacks" *very occasionally* is not a bad thing, but sometimes, especially at pancake houses, the cakes are the size of wagon wheels. That's where you must be careful to draw the line and stop when you know you've really had enough -- even if half the stack is still there! President Richard Nixon had a paranoia problem, but he was correct when he opined that the best exercise for keeping your weight down is pushing your chair back from the table. With pancakes, you definitely need to do that!

Of course, there are times, especially when traveling, that eating the breakfast you really should eat might not be possible. For example: When my wife and I have been in Scotland, we have often been served a "traditional Scottish breakfast." This layout of food is so iconic that the Scots even sell postcards with pictures of it. To many people, it looks disgusting, but nutritionally it packs a wallop and, whenever we have had it, we go the entire day on it, bypassing lunch altogether, and not eating anything again until evening. It consists of: a couple of eggs (any style), two sausages, a slice of tomato, a pile of baked beans, a piece of haggis (various organ meats ground up, heavily spiced and stuffed into a sleeve made of sheep intestine), a mushroom cap, and three slices of bacon. After consuming this, as I've said, you are good to go for at least eight hours. As for the haggis, don't knock it if you haven't tried it; it's my favorite part of the meal! If you lived in Scotland and ate this breakfast every day, you would weigh about 300 pounds unless you walked at least ten miles across the highlands each day . . . and drank no beer or Scotch! You may wonder why I include it in a book about diet and fitness. My answer: because you can eat foods loaded with protein and be so satisfied with all the nutrients you need for the day that you can go all the way to dinner without eating again and, if you *do* walk several miles across the highlands . . . or anywhere . . . you will not gain weight. You might very well lose some and be very fit.

So far, I haven't said a word about coffee. I think, with considerable scientific backing, that both coffee and tea are fine, possibly even beneficial. I drink a lot of coffee with milk in it . . . no sugar! If you currently *do* put sugar in your coffee, try to wean yourself off it. In the past, I always put sugar in coffee – couldn't imagine drinking it without it – but I gradually cut it back, eventually to zero. Now, coffee with sugar tastes grossly sweet. I did the same with salt. When my blood pressure started to show signs of rising, I began buying "low sodium" versions of soups and "V8" juice. At first, they tasted intolerably bland. But I gradually got used to them and now the "regular" soups and V8 taste so salty to me that I feel like I'm drinking sea water! So, you can do it, too: gradually cut out the sugar and salt that you may be addicted to.

So, that's it on breakfast. You may notice I don't even mention skipping it. That is a very bad idea! Starting the day with good nutrition, including plenty of protein, is essential. In my mind, the meal that can be skipped with no negative consequences is *lunch*.

LUNCH:

My Usual: As I said above, if I've had a "Scottish Breakfast" or even a particularly large bowl of oatmeal, I will eat a very small lunch or no lunch at all. Food is fuel, and if my tank isn't low, why fill it up just because the clock says 12:00? Of course, as I said above, I am not a food Nazi, so if you have a lunch meeting or a social reason to get together with people for lunch, or if you started your day at 5:00 A.M. and cannot possibly go to 6:00 P.M. without eating again, then, of course, do so. Just order or prepare something small, such as a salad. I often have a lunch meeting of the Kiwanis club I belong to, so I order a small cup of chili and I like the fact that I can converse more easily with the other people there because I don't always have my mouth stuffed with heavy food.

If I've had a small breakfast, lunch will be one of the following:

*a tuna salad and tomato sandwich

*a peanut butter and lettuce on whole wheat sandwich.
  Stop the fake gagging. It's good!

*a bowl of "Power Mix" vegetables

*a sliced ham or chicken sandwich.

*a salad of lettuce, tomato, carrots, cucumbers, Etc.
  Salad dressing: pear-infused vinegar (delicious; no mayo, no sugar)

There are many other possibilities for lunch. Just don't eat too much of anything! You pretty much can't go wrong if you eat moderately and avoid sugar. That means, of course, NO SOFT DRINKS AND NO DESSERT! The biggest killer of any weight control plan is sugar and there is hardly a dessert on the planet that doesn't feature sugar. I have gotten over the urge to eat an enormous lunch, topped off with a chocolate sundae. In the days when I *did* eat something like that, I would waddle off to try to be at my best the rest of the day and usually fail.

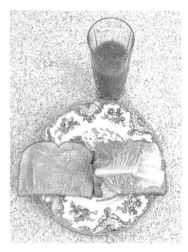

PB and lettuce ready for assembly. With a glass of vegetable juice, an excellent lunch

DINNER:

My Usual: To this day my children mock me for what they call my "Daddy dinner." On the two or three nights a week that my wife would be at work I would make dinner and it would always be some version of the same thing: a piece of meat (chicken breast, hamburger patty, hot dogs, fish sticks), mashed potatoes and a vegetable. I would always put as moderate sized portion of each item on their plates and not offer seconds. Occasionally, for variety, I would make spaghetti with meat sauce. As mock worthy as those meals were, they were well-balanced, and the little people who ate them are now full grown, mature, healthy adults with their own children. As far as I know, they have not endured any long-lasting maladies suffered because of the boring food I gave them. Furthermore, they are now serving up their own versions of the "daddy dinner" to their children.

By the way, if you are the cook, be careful how much tasting you do. In those days when I was the cook, I noticed myself practically eating a whole meal by sampling everything I was cooking. The calories can add up! Also, do not eat between meals -- granola bars, or anything else! You may think you need something, but the fact is, you don't! Keep carrots or celery around to munch if you simply must "munch" at 3 PM.

I thought when I got to "dinner" I'd have a lot to say about *what* to eat, but I really don't. I do have much to say about portion sizes. Portion control is important, especially with the bread and other starches. I would support eating more than you probably need of vegetables. They are pretty much a "freeby" as far as weight control is concerned . . . as long as they aren't slathered in great amounts of butter. If you want a mentally easy way to avoid overeating meat and mashed potatoes, keep munching on raw carrots, celery -- almost anything that would go into a salad.

If, half-way through the meal you are getting full... then stop eating!

Now, a very key point: If, half-way through the meal you are getting full and you can tell you have taken in enough "fuel," *then stop eating*! There are great containers available to save the leftovers for dinner tomorrow or tomorrow's lunch. When my wife and I eat at a restaurant, we almost always ask for a container to take home the extra food.

Very often the "extra" is enough for another meal the next night. You have to be superannuated to remember this, but it used to be you'd have to pretend you had a dog at home and tell the waiter you'd like a "doggy bag" to take the extra food home in. There was a famous cartoon in which the parents at a restaurant have clearly just asked the waiter for a" doggy bag" and their excited little boy, to his parent's total embarrassment, pipes up, "We're getting a dog!? "Imagine having to be surreptitious about eating sensibly and wanting to save food and money by taking home the extra food!

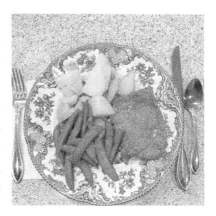

A typical "daddy dinner"

Then there is, once again, the matter of dessert. My advice is simple: Don't have any!

If your response is, "OK, Now You ARE being a food Nazi!" I say, try to be satisfied with something a little less egregious than a thick slice of chocolate cake or blueberry pie. I, too, crave sugar sometimes at the end of a meal and I have found an answer that isn't quite as satisfying as we might like, but it helps: stock up on Hershey's Chocolate kisses. I like the dark chocolate types, but any will do. They are only twenty calories a piece, so eat 2-3 of those. You get a taste of chocolate, and you leave the table happy! Well . . .sort of.

By the way, don't be a self-righteous jerk about any of this! If you are a guest at someone's house -- especially your mother's or mother-in-law's -- and she offers dessert, for goodness' sake have some, ask for another piece, and praise it! Don't ever self-righteously say "I'm watching my weight" or "I'm on a diet." Most people don't give a rat's ass that you're on a diet and, especially if they've spent hours preparing a dessert for you, they are annoyed when you tell them about your diet and wave away their beautiful creation.

Finally, I haven't said anything about drinking alcohol. On that, I have one rather serious confession. Many afternoons at 6:00 I relax with a glass of beer and some roasted almonds and watch the news. Can you control your weight and stay in shape if you have a beer every day? My answer is, you can if you do everything I have said about food and that I will say about exercise. It would be better not to drink alcohol at all, but if you (we) must do so, limit it to one drink per day. You can "get away with it" if you keep the exercise up.

So, that's about it on the food side of this very simple "plan." The mantra is "Eat less," (and avoid sugar). Your body needs a lot less fuel (food) than you think it does, so don't weigh it down and clog up the machinery with a lot of excess stuff!

Don't be self-righteous! Most people don't give a rat's ass that you're on a diet.

CHAPTER TWO

WALK MORE

Many people hate even hearing the term "exercise regimen." It conjures up images of super fit hard bodies wearing little tight-fitting outfits to accentuate their buffness and smiling while they do routines (weightlifting, bicycle pedaling, running) . . . routines that look an awful lot like work -- sweaty, fatigue-inducing, work. Furthermore, that work leaves "fitness freaks" exhausted and with no paycheck to show for their efforts. In fact, if they are at the gym or, much worse, paying a personal trainer, they finish not only more tired, but also poorer than when they started. No wonder Mark Twain said, "When I feel the urge to exercise, I lay down and rest until the urge goes away."

SIMPLE FITNESS

Advertising for exercise programs reaches the height of absurdity when a TV ad shows gullible viewers some new contraption guaranteed to bring its user hours of enjoyment and elevate his or her level of fitness to new heights! The film shows some paid actor smiling as he or she moves the levers or walks up phony stairs or does whatever the silly thing makes its user do. The ad assures viewers that they will want to do this over and over, every day, for the rest of their lives! Fat chance! This is all such a joke! Ninety-nine percent of the people who are gullible enough to purchase these machines will stop using them after they are bored to tears. Usually six weeks will do it. They will put their silly machine on eBay and go right on being out of shape and fighting to keep their weight down because they can't limit their calorie intake to less than what they consume in food every day.

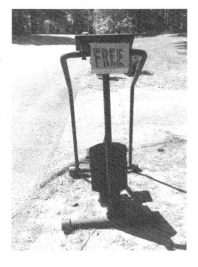

Then, there is bicycling. That form of exercise violates my basic principle: Keep it simple! The expense and headaches of the gear involved, and the time it takes to do a decent workout, disqualify it instantly as an exercise routine that a person will keep up for a lifetime. Well, I suppose it could be for a lifetime if the cyclist gets whacked from behind by the sideview mirror of a passing truck! I'm sounding terribly prejudiced here, but really -- an exercise routine that requires a helmet, an expensive bike that stops your workout cold when it breaks down, special shoes and fancy clothes, has within it far too many complications to be a lifetime fitness habit.

What makes this all very sad is that the way to avoid all that frustration and expense is absurdly simple: WALK! Just walk! Walk a lot and you will be in better shape than you are now and probably lose weight. Walk even more and you will be in even better shape. Walking is the best exercise there is! It is low-impact and can be performed almost anywhere with absolutely no equipment needed. Throw in a few push-ups and planks, do it every day, and you could very well get to be almost as buff looking and as fit as those hard bodies advertising absurd exercise machines. And all without traveling to a gym -- or a swimming pool, I might add -- or spending a dime on expensive equipment

Probably the most famous walking advocate was President Harry Truman. Every morning he drove the Secret Service guys and the press corps crazy as he walked at a very brisk pace from the White House, or wherever he happened to be. In his army days he had learned the 120 step per minute cadence, and that's what he did on his morning outings. He walked at least two miles each morning, leaving a sweating press corps in his wake, and after that he was good to start the day. He wore his business suit on these walks -- no need for a sweatsuit or running shoes -- and he was ready to head into the office the minute he walked through the door. As a man of few words and no need to pontificate on anything, he simply said that walking engages all the muscles in your body and gets your heart pumping faster. The

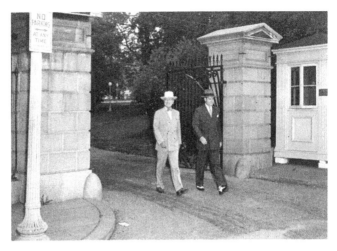

President Truman (white hat) out for his walk with a secret service agent. His advice: "Walk briskly, as if you are late for the meeting."

fresh air and exercise put you in a good frame of mind, and you are ready to "give 'em hell." The American people just thought of these walks as part of Truman's quirky personality. It's too bad everyone didn't follow his example and try to get as trim and fit as he was.

Probably the most common reason people give me for why they cannot walk or run every day is that they don't have the time. Well, if the President of the United States could find the time, we certainly can. Truman walked at 5:30 in the morning. That was always my choice, as well, because there was almost never anything else scheduled then. Of course, it was hard to get up an hour earlier than almost everyone else in town, but I got used to it and, after a few months, on a day when I didn't get out for a run, I

If the President of the United States could find the time, we certainly can.

felt irritable. Alternatively, some friends of mine have made walking at lunchtime their plan. That's fine -- except on those days, that happen all too often, when an unforeseen problem comes up that you must deal with. Then, there's the inverse of the early morning walk -- walking at night after everything is done -- all the kids are in bed, etc. I've tried that and it has the advantage of making you feel mellow when you head to the bedroom, but just like any other time of day, it competes with other things that other people might want to do at that time. The over-all answer to the problem is that you must make your walk a top priority and make it clear to everyone (including yourself) that somehow it is going to happen every day! You *will* walk *at least* two miles every day. End of story!

If I were to have written this ten years ago, or earlier, I would have advocated running or at least jogging, not walking. But, ever since I got "atrial fibrillation," I have not been able to run or jog -- at least not for very long -- and I have had to settle for walking. What I have discovered is that walking accomplishes the same things as running; it just takes a little longer. A four-mile run "back in the day" used to take me 30 minutes. Now, a four-mile walk takes me over an hour. So, I adjust my schedule to the new reality and still achieve the same results.

There are even a few positive differences that I experience from walking. I get less sweaty, especially in the cool weather so, if necessary, I can go right to an event, a meeting or whatever, without taking a shower. Also, I don't experience as many annoying little pains in ankles, knees or hips. And I am more inclined to get thoughtful and enjoy the scenery when I am not working hard to move fast.

And one more thing: I can relax and not feel competitive. I have enough things to feel competitive about without adding my recreational activity to the list. I used to enter road races and set high goals for myself, such as breaking three hours in the marathon. The first time I achieved that I was literally sobbing with relief and fatigue stretched out in the back seat of the car while my poor wife, Diane, drove me home from Boston. Today, I can come in from a five-mile walk relaxed, ready to have breakfast and eager to start the day.

In the "Eat Less" section I might have said, but didn't, that I cannot remember a single delicious meal I've ever eaten. By contrast, I remember many runs or walks I have truly enjoyed. Rather than bore you with descriptions that would mean something only to me, I will offer just one as a token example of so many runs or walks I have experienced. In California, I once took a run up a mountain in Oakland, circled the parking lot at the top and ran downhill on a long, winding road that offered spectacular views of San Francisco Bay and the Golden Gate Bridge. That happened over fifty years ago, but I still remember vividly the exhilaration I felt as I rounded each turn and got another panoramic view of the bay and the bridge shrouded in morning fog. It's my "go-to" memory for feeling mellow. I urge you to create your own memories of beautiful walks you have taken!

People sometimes ask, "How can I tell how far I've walked? Should I get a GPS watch?" My answer: No! No need for gimmicks. As far as step counting devices are concerned, I have little use for them, either. I can't count the steps I took going from the couch to the refrigerator for a beer the same as the steps I took walking up a hill on my favorite outdoor

walk! The alternative to GPS watches and step counters, is (as usual!) very simple! Measure a few routes around your area with your car. For variety, I sometimes go to an unfamiliar area to walk, and all I do is look at my watch when I start and assume I've gone a mile every time twenty minutes have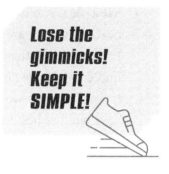
passed. My moderate walking pace is 18 minutes per mile, so even if I've stopped to view the scenery once or twice, I know I've walked a mile for each twenty minutes I've been out. The exact distance will not be precise, but does that matter?! Could it be any simpler than "I walked sixty minutes; I covered about three miles?" KEEP IT SIMPLE!! You may be able to walk a mile in fifteen minutes, or even less. Great! Adjust your calculations accordingly!

Many people who enjoy walking advocate listening to music or lectures with headphones on. If that's you, I have no problem with it, especially if it gets you out the door to hear what happens next in the book you are listening to. I don't use such devices because I'd rather use the time to think about issues, to pray, or to enjoy the scenery. Also, ever since a cross-country athlete in Chelmsford was killed by a train locomotive that he didn't hear, I've had an aversion to wearing anything that blocks my hearing of what is going on in my immediate environment. If you wear earpieces or headphones, please remember you are depriving yourself of one of the major ways you can sense impending danger.

What shoes are best? The answer is, of course, simple: Any shoe that's comfortable. I still buy running shoes (out of habit, or try to delude myself into thinking I'm still a "runner"), but there are dozens of walking shoes available from L.L.Bean and other outlets and, even just any old shoes you find comfortable and that don't give you blisters are perfectly fine. Truman wore wing-tipped dress shoes! Personally, I have had the best luck with Brooks running shoes or, lately, Hokas. When I first tried on Hokas I thought they were *too* cushioned, and I felt as if I were up on pillows. But I gradually got used to them and now they are my favorite brand.

When I'm about to start a walk, and after I finish, I always do a few stretchers. I've never been a stretching fanatic, even when I was a runner, so I don't spend a lot of time on it. Frankly, I find it a boring nuisance, but it is probably a good idea. A few toe touchers and wall leans and I'm ready. I think it's more important to start walking slowly and gradually pick up the pace during the first mile. After fifteen or twenty minutes you should feel more fluid, and your stride should be a little longer and you're in the groove. For the walk to do you the most good, you should keep the pace vigorous without "overstriding" or doing anything awkward that might strain a muscle or ligament, but don't start out too fast. Your goal is to get and stay fit, not be laid up with a muscle pull or debilitating hip or knee pain.

I often top off a vigorous walk with a set of push-ups and/or planks. As I've made pretty clear by now, I think it is best to work out with as little equipment as possible. Push-ups and planks require zero equipment. (A "plank" is simply holding yourself in push-up position -- back straight and level to the floor, abdominal muscles tightened for a length of time, at least thirty seconds A good, "varsity level "plank is held for two minutes.) Another good post-walk or post-run exercise is jumping jacks. When I coached, I shouted to the jumping high school kids that the soldiers in both world wars trained for storming the beaches with jumping jacks (check the old films). We were undefeated in world wars, so the "jacks" must have worked! All these post-walk strength exercises take, at most, ten minutes, and I only do them on alternate days. You can add sit-ups into the mix. I haven't done a sit-up since 2004 when I got a herniated disk in my back and found that sit-ups seemed to make it worse. My abs get strengthened in the walk and in the planks, so I'm "jacked" as much as I care to be "jacked." For most of us, developing impressive muscles is not the priority. The goal is to be trim, stay healthy, feel good and have a positive outlook on life. A vigorous walk and a set of push-ups and planks will put you in a good place mentally, at least once you get used to it.

Now, an important point: You may want or *need* to start out with very low expectations -- say a half-mile walk around the block, a small number of push-ups or jacks -- until you have built up your endurance. I'm a huge advocate of "easing into" anything -- a hard job or an exercise routine. Start easy; save the hard stuff for when you are ready for it.

Another important point: You will stay with this and get and stay fit for the rest of your life if you think of it as *fun*. Get friends and/or family members to go with you -- not every day, but maybe once a week. Find new places to walk, even if it means driving to another town. And DO NOT do what a friend of mine did several years ago when he tried to start a running program. He set up a one-mile loop and covered it every morning, each day trying to beat his time from the previous day. When he got to the point when he was unable to do his "personal best," he quit. I told him to stop *timing* himself at all and to have fun; make it be the one thing he did each day in which he did not have to compete or excel. He said he was simply too competitive to do it that way. He stopped exercising and went on to become a big fat guy who had a lot of money and drove a huge Cadillac. I don't know if he's happy; I doubt it.

> **Start with low expectations and make it FUN!**

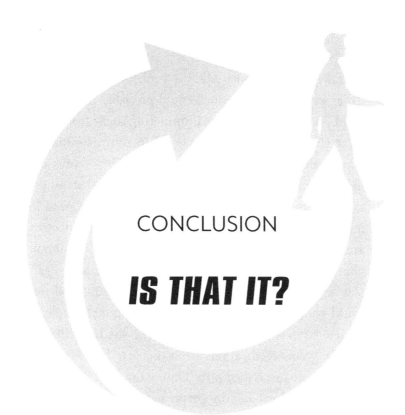

CONCLUSION

IS THAT IT?

The short answer to the question is "Yes!" The answer to the question "How can I lead a healthy life and control my weight?" is extremely simple: Eat less; walk more! But like so many other things in life, it is simple . . . but not easy. I'll say it again: "easy" and "simple" are not synonyms.

So, how does one prepare oneself to "simply" eat less and walk more? Let me suggest three important paradigm changes that you must make if you are going to successfully adopt my lifestyle plan. I have alluded to these already; now I will flat out say them.

1. Think of food as fuel for your body to give it the energy it needs, and medicine for your body to prevent and/or cure illness. The "medicine" part of the sentence above it not a mistake or a hyperbole. Many -- probably most -- of the drugs people are prescribed could probably be replaced by important diet changes. Eliminating sugar from their diets would keep many people off insulin; eliminating excess salt would help many people get off blood pressure medications. The mindset we have today is that we get sick because diseases just happen to us and we need to take medications to fight them. As I stated earlier, doctors are even starting to prescribe drugs to counter childhood obesity! Nonsense! Children should just eat less sugar, play actively, and NOT GET fat! In this country, if not world-wide, we have developed a pill popping lifestyle. If someone has a physical ailment, he or she immediately thinks, "What medications are available to fix this?" I am against over-prescribed pills. Unlike the pharmaceutical companies I don't stand to make a dime if people adopt my way of thinking about their health. Our country -- indeed the entire world -- could save billions in medical costs if people would simply eat the right foods in the right amounts and go for long walks!

2. Number "2" is a corollary to number "1." Except for trying to eat the right things for your health and physical well-being, do not make food the focus of your life. I can remember many wonderful meals but the memories *all* have to do with the people who were there and the environment we were sitting in -- the view, the charm of the room, etc. My memories of those meals have *nothing* to do with the food I ate. I can't even begin to remember what food I put into my mouth on any of those occasions.

Naturally, at a special gathering of family or friends, I appreciate at the time the good food and the effort that someone or several people put forth to prepare it. But, if the same people were there, I could be just as happy if the table featured a jar of peanut butter with a knife stuck in it and a bowl of crackers.

3. Think of your daily walk as fun, not a chore to be accomplished. It may seem like work at first, but once you adapt to it, you will look forward to your walk every day. There are villages in Britain where the people once gathered in the town square every Saturday morning to go for a group hike through the pastures and nearby forests. After an hour or two of brisk hiking, they gathered again at the church or town square for a communal breakfast. What a great tradition! And I hope it continues even as modern times have placed so many obstacles in the way of such a thing. If we adopted this tradition in our towns, think of the improvements in health, both physical and mental, we would see! Perhaps some churches today could adopt this activity to improve the health of their congregations. Just a thought. I hope someone will walk with it. I've been thrilled to see that several walking groups *have* started up in my hometown of Andover.

I never tire of touring on foot -- which is what walking really is. I always do a different route each day. Sometimes I go to the local "AVIS" (Andover Village Improvement Society) path and walk through the woods. Other days I will walk for an hour around the beautiful Phillips Academy campus. When we lived in Winchester, I even loved going for runs in urban settings. I often went to the Cambridge YMCA and ran around the city with a group of guys who started their runs at the "Y." One of the runners, a man named Manny Slate, owned a drug store in Cambridge, and nearly everyone in the city knew him. One day, as we ran down busy Mass Ave., a guy yelled out, "Hey Manny, how come ya runnin'? I don't see no cops!" We all chuckled a bit and waved to the guy as we weaved through the traffic. You see and meet many people on an urban run or walk and it's fun!

Every time we visit a new place, the first thing I want to do is take a run -- nowadays, a walk -- through the area. It is a great way to scope out the terrain, learn the streets, and start to meet the people.

In the final analysis, I think everyone would agree that my plan would improve their health IF they could adopt it and stick to it. There's the rub (as the Brits say), and that is what this concluding section has attempted to address. I hope I have convinced you that eating less and walking more is a good lifestyle plan.

Allow me one last pitch: A British actor named Dawn French starred in a sitcom called "The Vicar of Dibley," in which she played the first female vicar in a small English town. She was very funny and decidedly overweight. As the years progressed, she trimmed down noticeably (probably by as much as one hundred pounds) and people were asking her how she did it. Her answer: I cut back on the amount of food I ate, and I went for long walks every day. She implied the walks were torture, but nevertheless she did them and the results were startling. So, there it is: She ate less, walked more, and lost one hundred pounds,.

However, I know there are people who feel they would be miserable living their lives the way I'm advocating. They love to eat and the idea of taking long walks every day -- and trying to fit them into their schedule -- is too annoying to contemplate. If that is you, and you are near the end of this polemic unconvinced and unwilling to at least give my lifestyle plan a try, I thank you for your attention (which has gotten you this far!) and I wish you well.

To those of you who already do most of what I've advocated here, I say "Hello, kindred spirits! I'm sure you have nodded in agreement to nearly everything I've said and could have added some helpful thoughts of your own. Carry on!"

Finally, to those readers who rarely exercise and eat carelessly but nevertheless are on board to give this a try, I say this: "Welcome! Good for you! Take the first steps. Buy the good foods and throw away the bad. Make sure you have the right shoes for walking. Pray for continued good health, think positive thoughts, decide you are going to enjoy your new life, and look forward eagerly to tomorrow morning when you will take a bracing walk, eat a healthy breakfast, and head out the door feeling positively blessed that you are alive!"

APPENDIX A

A SAMPLE HEALTHY DAY

EARLY MORNING: WALK (OR RUN, IF YOU CAN) 2-5 MILES; DO PUSH-UPS

Eat breakfast:
large bowl of oatmeal,
blueberries, banana
Or
Two eggs and whole wheat toast

NOON TIME: *Eat a light lunch:*
Salad with moderate amount of dressing
Or
Bowl of power mix vegetables
Or
Peanut butter and lettuce on whole wheat, or other moderately sized sandwich.

AFTERNOON:

(If you have a strong urge to snack: keep carrots, celery, etc in frig. ready to grab)

(If you are "the cook" for the evening, DO NOT FREQUENTLY TASTE TEST!).

DINNER: *Eat dinner of your choice:*
                       MODERATE PORTIONS!
                       No dessert . . . Or 3 Hershey's "kisses".

EVENING: If you haven't fit in a walk yet, do it *now*. Do not unnecessarily allow a day to go by without a walk!

Remember: If you are on the dark streets, drivers cannot see you unless you wear reflective clothing. You DO have the **right** to be on the street, but you don't want to be "**dead right!**"

APPENDIX B

A FEW FAQ OR COMMON COMMENTS

Why don't you discuss calories in this book?

I think calorie counting is just another complication we can do without. We all know that sugar, butter, beer and many other delights have many calories and that if we consume a great deal of those and don't exercise much, we will gain weight. Tabulating everything is an annoying bore, so I don't, and you shouldn't either. Just eat less and walk more and the numbers will take care of themselves.

SIMPLE FITNESS

You denounce gyms, exercise equipment and personal trainers, but don't those provide motivation and encouragement that many people need?

I suppose I'm straight out of the last century. After all, I refer to a guy who was president seventy years ago (Truman) as my prime example. But I believe many of the gimmicks we rely on these days have made us soft, not only physically but also mentally. We need to learn to be mentally strong and know that we can achieve fitness and good health without having to use expensive equipment or pay people $200 an hour to encourage us. I'll use a little "tough love" here: Don't be one of those pansies who needs machines and personal trainers!

I don't have a treadmill and don't want to spend a lot of money to buy one, so what should I do during a spell of bad weather?

In Scotland, home of my ancestors, they have an expression: "There's no bad weather, only bad preparation." If it's raining, put on a slicker; if it's cold, put on a coat and gloves. There are limits; you shouldn't venture out in a howling blizzard. But most of the time, you can handle the weather if you simply dress for it. I do have a treadmill, but I use it only when it would be truly unsafe to venture outside.

A jar of peanut butter and a bowl of crackers at a social gathering would satisfy you?! I really doubt it.

That was a bit of hyperbole, and I should have added that I would also want a cooler of beer on hand to go with the crackers and peanut butter. Yet, I stand by my point. I care much more about the people who are present than the food that is available.

You never mention yoga. Many people swear by that as a great exercise regimen. What are your thoughts on that?

Yoga does ring bells for many people, and they swear it increases their flexibility, is mentally soothing, and burns calories. I won't dispute those claims but, like stretching (which is what it really is) I find it boring and tedious. I prefer an exercise routine that is less static, and gets me out the door rather than sticks me indoors with a group of sweaty people. Also, I'm not convinced it improves cardio-vascular fitness or burns many calories.

What do you do if you sprain an ankle or break a leg and can't walk for six weeks or more?

This is a quandary that has always bedeviled people who want to stay physically fit. The first thing I'll say is that I never just sit around waiting for the lay-off time to be over. If the doctors allowed it, I would walk with the boot on or with crutches. If that were not possible (or even if it were possible) I would do as much upper body work with weights as I could. There is almost no excuse for becoming completely sedentary. If I were confined to a jail cell (on phony charges, of course!) I would run in place, do push-ups by the hundreds, do jumping jacks . . . in other words, do everything possible under the circumstances to stay fit. Never let anything short of being tied up or dead prevent you from keeping physically fit.

I really dislike just walking or running without a purpose. I agree with the guy who called out to your friend, "Why are you running? I don't see any cops." Listening to audio books would help motivate me a lot, yet you discourage that. Can you clarify your views?

I did offer cautionary advice about walking and listening to audio books, and I personally don't choose to do it, but many people find it truly enjoyable. To have your mind occupied by a worthwhile book (or podcast) makes the miles go by more easily. As long as you remember that you have to stay visually alert, then I would recommend it as a way to motivate yourself to get out the door. With apologies to my Audubon Society friends who hate this expression, you get to "kill two birds with one stone" -- enrich your mind while you exercise your body. Perhaps I should leave the birds out of this and simply say "it's a win-win activity."

What do you say to "foodies" who love food, love to cook and find most of what you recommend in the "Eat Less" chapter insulting and boring? They think your plan would suck all the joy out of life.

To "Foodies" I say this: If you adopt my approach to eating you only must exercise *portion control*! You are free to be as creative and flamboyant in your cooking as you wish.

My "go-to" culture for this concept is France. The French have botched many things: They never finish anything. They don't finish pronouncing their words (e.g. *Versailles;* what happens to the final "lles?"); they don't finish their wars (World War I, World War II, Vietnam. We had to finish up all of those for the French). BUT, what they have gotten right is food, especially portion control. In a fancy French restaurant, if you order a steak, you will get a lonely four ounce chunk of meat lost in the middle of an enormous plate, swimming in a delicious sauce and topped with a sprig of parsley. The presentation is a bit silly, but the concept of being satisfied with a minimal amount of truly delicious food is spot on. A book came out a few years ago titled *French Women Don't Get Fat: The Secret of Eating For Pleasure.*" One of the concepts in that book was that French women, when they cook, concentrate on quality rather than quantity. And that's what I say about food, "Quality rather than quantity." I'm very glad the U.S. saved the French in the world wars so they could continue to set us straight about how to eat.

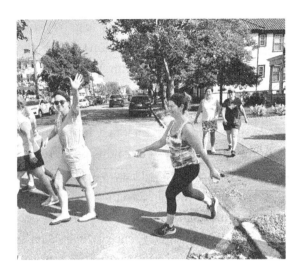

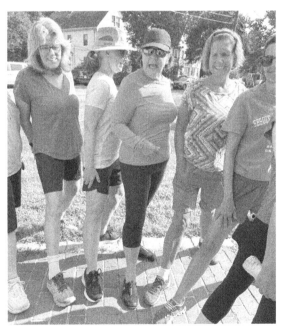

Thank You to Patti Longo (third from the right) and her group The Town Walkers for allowing me to photograph them for the cover photo and the ones seen above.

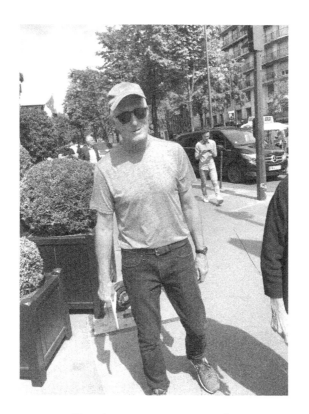

"Anywhere you are, you can walk."
Photo taken at Av. des Champs-Élysées, Paris

WA

Made in the USA
Monee, IL
22 February 2025

12576748R00030